Autism Awareness:

An Alarming Requirement

Autism and Life After 20 years

By

Dr. Anshul Saxena

© All Rights Reserved.2017

<u>Disclaimer</u>

No part of the book may be reproduced or transmitted in any form or by any means, mechanical or electronic including photocopying or recording or by any information storage and retrieval system or transmitted by e mail without permission in writing from the author and publisher. The views in the book are originally expressed by the author alone.

Contents

- Acknowledgement
- Introduction
- Autism Awareness : An Alarming Requirement
- What is Autism
- Signs and Symptoms
- Autism and Life After 20 years
- Conclusion : An Appeal
- About Author

Acknowledgement

First and foremost, I express my gratitude to the Almighty God who blessed me with thoughts, ideas, words and capability to pen down them on the paper. Without His blessings and inspiration, I would have never been able to write this book.

I would like to submit my heartiest gratitude to my husband and my child for their invaluable and constant support to complete my book.

I am deeply indebted to my

respected parents for being my constant supporters to encourage my writings. I also thank to my in-laws for their possible support.

    My joy knows no bounds in expressing my special thanks to my brother, sister and sister in law for their keen interest and precious advice.

__Introduction__

The progress of a country depends on various factors. As it is said, '*Health is Wealth*'. Physical and mental health of a country's citizens plays a very important role for the growth of that country.

There is an alarming rise in the number of children suffering with neuro-developmental disorder like Autism spectrum disorder. Statistics show there is a continuous increase in number of such kind of cases year by year.

This book is written to highlight AUTISM- its sign, symptoms and possible causes. Author of this book has tried to depict some imaginary consequences for autism after 20 years, in the absence of precautionary steps to control autism.

The author has tried her best to share her knowledge about autism to make people aware with Autism. The views expressed in this book are author's own thoughts based on her experience and observation in the field of Autism.

The following information, provided in this book, should not be used to diagnose or treat a child with autism. Symptoms, conditions and ways to deal a child, vary from child to child. A consultation or supervision by an experienced doctor or psychiatrist is always suggested.

(I)
Autism Awareness:

An Alarming Requirement

The progress of a country depends on various factors. As it is said, "Health is Wealth". Physical and mental health of a country's citizens plays a very important role for the growth of that country.

    Our country India is going to face a very serious problem regarding mental illness or mental disabilities. There is an alarming rise in the number of children suffering with neuro-developmental disorder like Autism spectrum disorder or autism. Autism Spectrum Disorder (ASD) is the name for a group of developmental disorders. ASD includes a wide range, "a spectrum", of symptoms, skills and levels of disability.

Statistics show there is a continuous increase in number of such kind of cases year by year.

India has about 10 million people with autism (the data can vary as many cases remain undiagnosed) and the disability has shown an increase over the last few years. Experts estimate that 1 in 66 children between ages 2 to 9 are affected with Autism in India against ratio 1 in 110 few years back. It has been observed that Autism is more common among the boys than the girls.

Though various causes for Autism spectrum disorder have been predicted in various theories yet no specific reason has been proved for being a child to be autistic. It is believed that Autism can be caused by genetic, environmental, immunological or metabolic factors. Statistics updates are being given frequently. Researches are on their ways. Different theories are being given. The exact cause for Autism is still unknown.

Health experts believe that the first sign usually appear in the first 3 years. Early detection can help a child lead his life with full potential if he is well attended with early intervention. As initial years are very important for a child's brain to grow, so the maximum work can be done with the child during formative years to get the best possible results. After that also the positive involvement to teach the child should be continued. A child can be provided with the required therapies like speech and language therapy or occupational therapy etc.

In India these symptoms like poor eye contact, self play, lack of verbal or nonverbal interaction, sensory overload, repetitive behaviour and stereotype pattern of behaviour, impairment in social interaction are either ignored by parents or undiagnosed or misdiagnosed by many medical professionals which is one of the major reasons for the higher numbers in the country.

April 2 is celebrated as WAAD i.e. World Autism Awareness Day, still a large number of people are unaware about the word autism. Media, the strongest medium for spreading information, does not focus to cover up any news or story about autism even on

Autism day. It never comes as headlines on news channels or in newspapers. Sometimes news about autism can be seen flashing in a column by a few news papers.

My concern to write this book about autism

is just to make people aware with autism and autism related issues so that some precautions can be taken on time to make the situation better. Seeing the alarming increase in the number of autistic kids, the more awareness should be spread in our country.

(II)
<u>Autism</u>

Autism is a neurodevelopmental disorder that causes a person's disability to communicate and relate to other people. Autism is known as 'spectrum disorder'. It first appears in young children, who fall along a spectrum from mild to severe. The term "spectrum" reflects the wide variation in challenges and strengths possessed by each person with autism. This word 'spectrum' describes the range of difficulties that people on the autism spectrum may experience and the degree to which they may be affected. Some people with autism may be able to live near normal lives independently while some may need lifelong support. Some may have exceptional abilities some may not.

Medically, autism is considered as a lifelong developmental disability.

Wikipedia defines, "Autism is a neuro-developmental disorder characterized by impaired social interaction, verbal and nonverbal communication and restricted and repetitive behaviour."

Autistic people whether children or adults have difficulty to have eye contact with other persons. They prefer to be in their own world. They have difficulty to learn socially appropriate behavior. They have very different way to observe the things which can sometimes be beyond our imagination. On one hand, If they have some limitations, they can have some strength in particular field on the other hand. If their strength is noticed and worked upon on proper time, miracles cannot be unobserved.

Autism is a state of being different-different from neuro typical person. Each autistic person is a different individual. Many symptoms can be similar but there cannot be any comparison between two autistic persons.

(III)

<u>Signs and Symptoms for Autism</u>

Autism's most-obvious signs tend to appear between 2 and 3 years of age. Some children show signs from birth. Other children seem to grow normally but suddenly by the age of 18 to 36 months, the symptoms appear.

With careful observation and under the supervision and guidance of an experienced person or a doctor, autism can be detected at very early age.

Early signs for autism may include:

- The child does not have eye to eye contact.
- The child doesn't turn to his mother's voice.
- The child does not respond to his own name.
- He has no babbling or finger pointing by age of one.

- There may be no smile or respond to others who try to communicate verbally or non-verbally.
- They may have unusual responses to people, attachments to objects, resistance to change in their routines, or aggressive or self-injurious behavior.

- At times they may seem not to notice people, objects, or activities in their surroundings.
- These children may find it hard to have *joint attention*. That means a child may seem either taking no interest when adults point out objects, such as a car running

on the road or he may show no interest to catch others attention to show them the same thing of his interest.

The core symptoms for autism can be observed in the following areas.

(i)Difficulties in Social Communication and Social Interaction

Autistic people face difficulty to develop verbal or non verbal communication skills. They may find it difficult to use or understand facial expressions, body posture, jokes, *sarcasm* and tone of voice. They may avoid eye contact. Some children may have delay in learning to talk while few children with autism may not develop speech at all or may have limited speech. They find it easier to understand what is said to them than to express what they want to say to others. They take time to process what is said to them. Sometimes they repeat the words, phrases or sentences said by another person that is called 'echolalia'.

They have lack of empathy and may find it difficult to understand another person's feelings like pain or sorrow and to express their own feelings. It is difficult for them to read others intentions.

 They can have problem to understand implied meaning or humour as they interpret word for word meaning said by another person. They may struggle to understand *abstract* concepts.

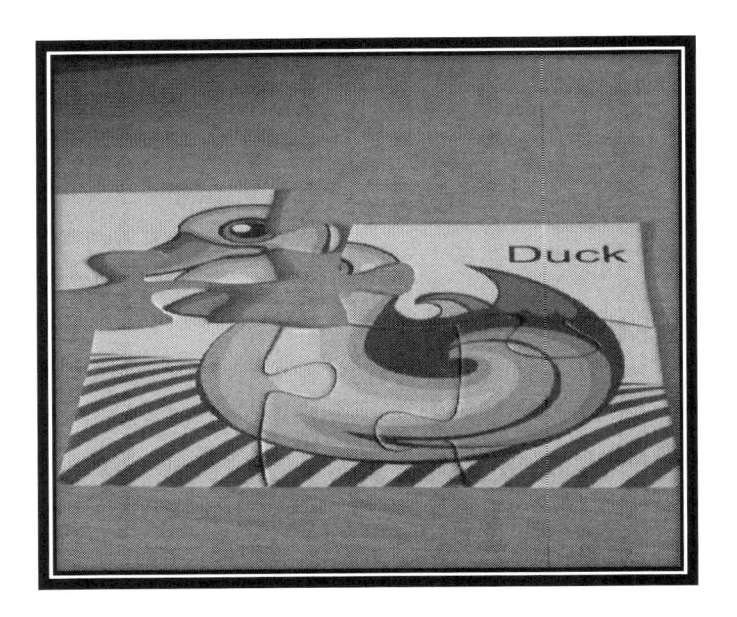

They may find it hard to make friends as they face problem to interact or to understand the way to form friendship.

(ii)Restricted and repetitive patterns of behaviours, activities or interests:

A child with autism looks just like any other

child, but has distinctive behavior patterns.

That child may often prefer to have a daily routine so that he knows what is going to happen every day. He may have a need for sameness and routines. For example he may insist you to follow the same route to go to the shopping mall or he may always listen to particular music while having evening snacks.

People with autism may feel uncomfortable with sudden change in their routine but they can cope with that change, if they are prepared for that change in advance. Uncertain change without prior information or preparation can be a reason for their anxiety.

It may be difficult for an autistic person to

take a different approach to something once they have been taught the 'right' way to do it. It is more difficult for autistic people to 'unlearn' something they have learnt before.

Stereotyped behaviours:

Children who are autistic may have *stimming* or repetitive and stereotyped behaviours such as rocking, pacing, spinning, head movement, finger waving, or hand flapping. In this condition a child may have repetitive body movements or repetitive movement of objects.

Symptoms may include a child's **limited interests in activities or play**. An autistic toddler does not seem to be interested in playing certain games, such as peek-a-boo.

A child with autism may have an unusual focus on pieces or objects which are not toys. Younger children with autism often focus on parts of toys, such as the wheels on a car, rather than playing with the entire toy. They may have limited pretend play.

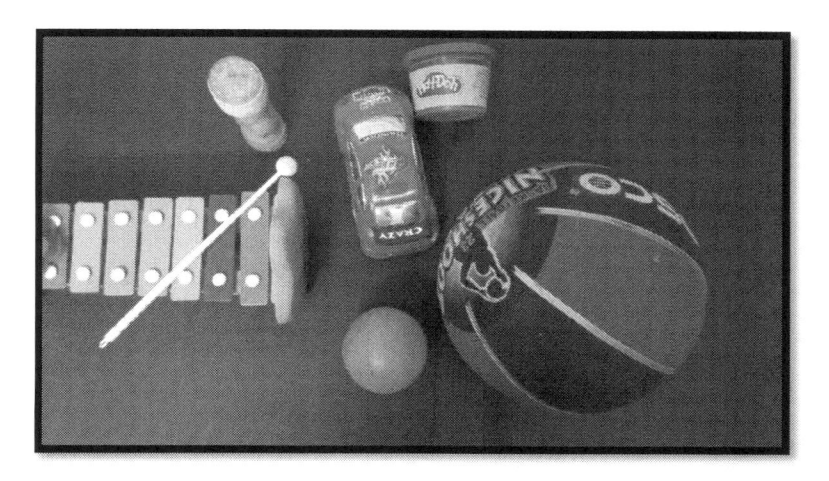

Sometimes the child may move very quickly from one activity to another and may appear to be hyper active.

Other Signs and Symptoms

Children with autism sometimes may have physical symptoms like some may have digestive problems such as constipation .They may have sleep problems like sleeping for few hours or sleeping very late at night. Such children may feel very fresh by taking a short nap or sometimes they may feel very drowsy the whole day because of uncertain sleeping pattern. Children may have poor coordination of the large muscles used for running and climbing, or the smaller muscles of the hand. About a third of people with autism may also have seizures or mental retardation.

Highly-focused interests

Many autistic people may have intense and highly-focused interests since their childhood. That interest can be anything like art, music, mathematics, science or computers. Their interest may change over time or it can remain lifetime.

Sensory Sensitivity

Children with autism may experience over- or under- sensitivity to sounds, touch, tastes, smells, light, colours, temperatures or pain similar to a condition known as sensory processing disorder. For example, they may get agitated or may not bear certain background sounds, which are ignored or unnoticed by other people. They may be captivated by lights or spinning objects.

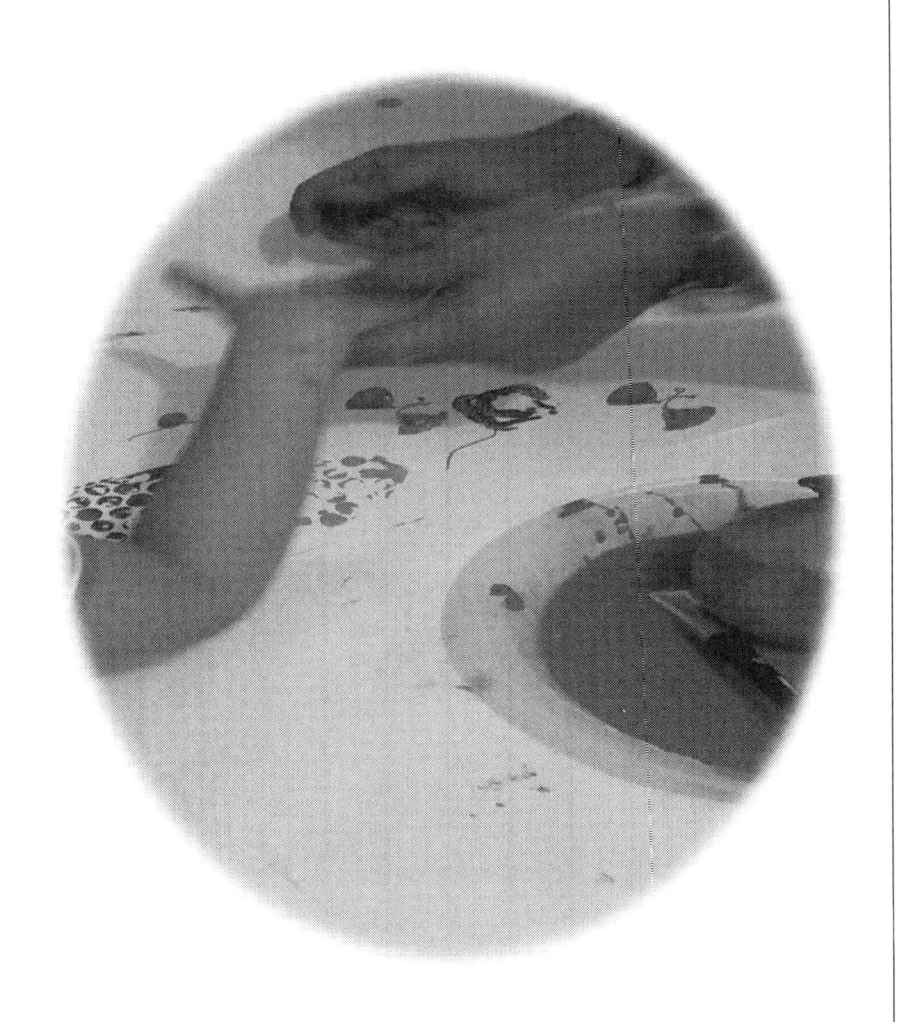

Autistic children with sensory sensitivity may

have the following other symptoms.

- They may be excessively sensitive to sounds like pressure cooker's whistle; car's horn or sound by mixer grinder.
- They may have difficulty handling small objects such as buttons.

- They may like jumping, swinging or spinning excessively.
- They may have difficulty to chew certain foods.
- They may be hypersensitive to certain fabrics and only wear clothes that are soft or comfortable.

- They may be oversensitive to some particular smells or odors like perfumes, moisturizer or any cream.
- They may dislike getting their hands or face dirty.

- Some of them may not like to be touched or held by others.

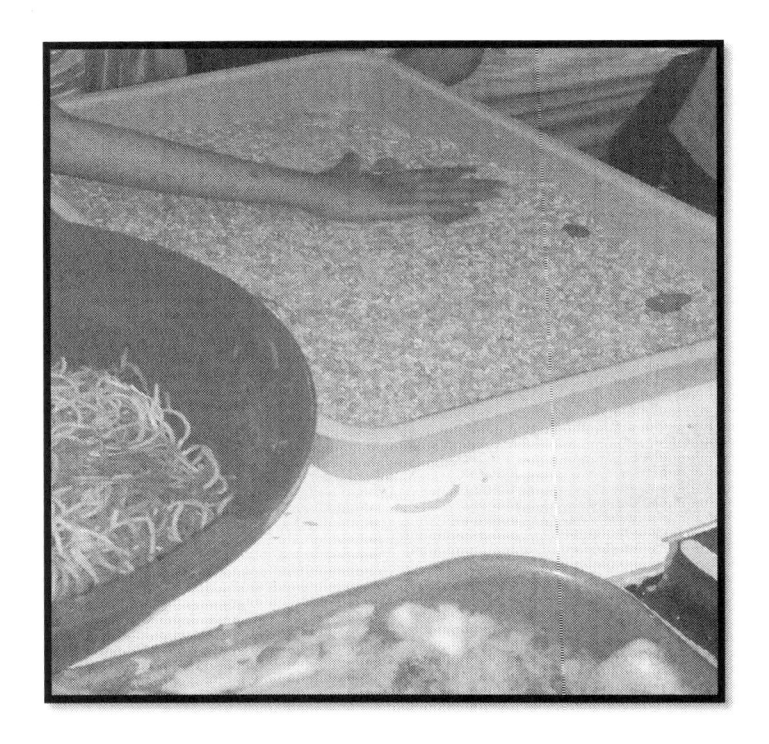

All these symptoms related to sensory sensitivity can be treated by sensory integration therapy. This recommended therapy is usually conducted by an occupational or physical therapist.

(IV)
Autism and Life after 20 Years

There is dramatic increase in the cases of mental disorders or intellectual disabilities. The way number of autistic kids is increasing, is quite surprising and alarming too. Several years back, only a few autism cases were observed but the shocking fact is this that the ratio of autistic kids is increasing every year. We hardly hear any news about autism recovery. If this situation will not be controlled who will support whom?

    Though several reasons, causes, signs and symptoms for autism have been found out but exact reason or proper cure for autism could not be invented yet. Although, researches are being done to find out the exact cause and cure, the result is still awaited since years.

  Has anybody imagined if proper cure could not be found on time or autism could not be controlled, what will our country be like after 20 years?

Seeing the alarming boost in autism cases, I just imagined our country after 20 years.

At present many people are not even acquainted with the word autism. They are completely unaware about it. But in future, it will not be so. People will not only be aware with this disorder but they will also have autistic people in their neighbor, friend circle or may be in their family because of the increasing number of autism cases.

As many autistic people can lead their life in a better way, if they have some structured schedule for their routine work.

Considering their need, such kind of institutions or apartments can be constructed in future.

I think Autistic people will have their own societies or apartments in future, where neuro-typical people (normal people in common words) will look different to them.

Many autistic people are very good at mathematics. They can calculate like a calculator. They do not know to lie or cheat. So very soon in future, companies will prefer autistic people to hire for the post of accountant or any other post.

It can also be possible that autistic people have their own work places where special seats will be reserved for autistic persons.

There comes a time when particular courses in education are in demand. I will not be surprised, if a demand arises for the course in special education in coming years. I think Special Education will be introduced in all the colleges and institutions as it will be a dire need to understand special people. At present, very few people (mostly parents of autistic kids) opt for special education diploma or other courses in special education. No wonder, if in future students choose courses in special education as better career option for job placement.

Have you imagined what will be our

education system in coming years? At present, parents of an autistic child are struggling to get him admitted in a school. Schools have very limited seats for special children in their school. They do not have efficient and trained teachers to deal with special children.

As the number of these children is growing so rapidly, in future instead of limited seats the number of seats for special children may increase in the schools.

It may be possible that every section of class rooms has special children.

Autistic children can learn very fast and perform in an excellent manner, if they are taught the way they learn. It may be possible that special curriculum is introduced for these children the way they learn. It may have separate course books for them.

It may be possible that it becomes compulsory for the teachers to do a special course and training to deal and teach special children.

As we see reserved seats for woman, physically disabled or old people in the public transport, in future we will see reserved seats for special persons

(Intellectually Disabled) also.

We can have special arrangements for special people at shopping complex or market places. People will be more tolerant and understanding for disabled persons.

Few positive results, I can imagine with the increasing number of autistic persons that there will also be augmentation of honesty, truthfulness, faithfulness, pure love and affection in relationships. At some places there will be accuracy in work without any hypocrisy and diplomacy.

    Everything mentioned above in this part of the

book, is surely something nobody would like to see in future. It can just be a bitter consequence, if precautions are not taken.

(V)
Conclusion: An Appeal

In the end, I would like to make an appeal that we should try to make people aware about autism spectrum disorder at our level best. Autism awareness is really an alarming requirement. There is nothing to hide. The more is shared the more would be cared.

Everybody should understand that autism is not a contagious disease. It is not spread by touching or coming in contact with autistic person. Autistic people also have right to education, right to equality, right against exploitation or right to live in the society. They may have some limitations but they should be provided opportunities. They should not be left unheard, unattended or underestimated.

If a person has weak eyes and can see clearly with the help of glasses, it does not mean that he cannot do the things what others can do. In the same way, autistic people need support to do better in their life. If God has made us capable of helping others, we should always be ready for that to make our life worth living.

About Author

The author of this book, **Dr.Anshul Saxena** has keen interest and passion for writing. She has written many articles, several poems and blogs. She has been writing since years. She is a blogger, writer, a poet and now an author and publisher also. She has written and published other books also.

Books by **Dr. Anshul Saxena:**

- Autism: Signs, Symptoms, Causes. 8 Important Tips to Improve Autistic Children
- Secrets of Successful and Happy Life
- Success Mantra: A Short Story

- How to Speak In English: Very Useful Tips
- Self Improvement: Know Your Potential

Three story books below have been written for sight reading. These will be very good books for special and other kids as well to enhance their reading abilities.

3. A Day with Mary: A Guessing Game Story

4. 7 Days and Mary's Activities

5. Good Habits: Peter Got a Lesson

Contact:

exploremoreandlearn@gmail.com

Printed in Great Britain
by Amazon